Not Superwomen

12-Month Nutrition Planner

Shekema Sims

ISBN: 978-0-578-84440-4

Published by Shekema Sims

Edited by Ready Writer Services LLC

Introduction

My name is Shekema Sims! If you're familiar with my *Not Superwomen* physical fitness guide, then you already know I love working out! But I'm sure you can agree that sometimes gyms and personal trainers can be over your budget and overwhelming, depending on what season you're in. And, when we're moms of little ones, it can be tough to find childcare so we can go to the gym or time to plan out healthy meals. This is where I was! I started working out after I had my second child and had put on some unwanted weight. But I couldn't afford a personal trainer and my kids were too small to stay home alone.

Still, I was determined! So, I got an elliptical machine from my grandmother and started working out 20 minutes a day, 3 times a week. Because I was a mom of little kids, I had to be strategic with my workout schedule. I had to work out before the kids got up. Three times a week, I'd set my alarm for 6:00 am. I also had to be strategic with my meals and mealtimes. I needed to change not just in my physical activity but also in what I was putting in my body! The hardest part for me was drinking water because it wasn't a beverage I liked. But putting these things together was the best move I had made for myself!

Then, as my health journey continued, I started thinking about other women. Women just like me. I started asking myself how I could help them achieve their fitness goals. How could I help them feel better about themselves? What can I do to help women who live busy lives but want to also live healthy lives? To help them realize that even in the busyness of life, motherhood, marriage, work, and everything else; they can exercise and eat right.

So, I started with the *Not Superwomen:* Physical Fitness Guide and it has made working out so much easier for women and less intimidating. But, then I developed the *Not Superwomen 12-Month Nutrition Planner*! And this planner is everything I wish I had when I started my fitness journey! This planner not only has a monthly calendar for you to jot down appointments or any personal life events; it also has a place for you to set your goals, track your victories, plan your meals, and schedule them. In fact, you can even write your groceries as you map out your health goals!

Remember, this isn't about doing a whole 180 degree turn over night. This is about creating a healthy lifestyle that will last! It's about taking the necessary steps to change your mindset on fitness and building from there! Ladies, we are Not Superwomen in that we don't have to be everything to everyone to the point of leaving ourselves behind! But we are super in that we can make the choice to change our lives for better each day! You can do this!

I'd love to be a part of your continued healthy lifestyle journey! For further exercise routines or nutritional consultations, contact me:

Email: shekemasims@yahoo.com

OR

Phone: 856-655-1991

Follow me on Facebook @lifestylenotadiet

and Instagram @notsuperwomen

JANUARY

Sunday	Monday	Tuesday	Wednesday	Thursday	Friday	Saturday
					1	2
3	4	5	6	7	8	9
10	11	12	13	14	15	16
17	18	19	20	21	22	23
24	25	26	27	28	29	30
31						

WEEKLY GOALS!
1.
2.
3.
4.

WORKOUT SCHEDULE

	M	T	W	Th	F	S	S
Week 1	am pm	am pm	am pm	am pm	am pm	am pm	am pm
Week 2	am pm	am pm	am pm	am pm	am pm	am pm	am pm
Week 3	am pm	am pm	am pm	am pm	am pm	am pm	am pm
Week 4	am pm	am pm	am pm	am pm	am pm	am pm	am pm

Goal Tracker!

Weight	Non-scale Victories

Monthly Meal Planner

Grocery List

Meal Planning

Breakfast

1.
2.
3.
4.

Lunch

1.
2.
3.
4.

Dinner

1.
2.
3.
4.

Snacks

1.
2.
3.
4.

Meal Tracker

M	T	W	Th	F	S	S
6 a - 10 a	6 a - 10 a	6 a - 10 a	6 a - 10 a	6 a - 10 a	6 a - 10 a	6 a - 10 a
11 a - 2 p	11 a - 2 p	11 a - 2 p	11 a - 2 p	11 a - 2 p	11 a - 2 p	11 a - 2 p
3 p - 4 p	3 p - 4 p	3 p - 4 p	3 p - 4 p	3 p - 4 p	3 p - 4 p	3 p - 4 p
5 p -8 p	5 p -8 p	5 p -8 p	5 p -8 p	5 p -8 p	5 p -8 p	5 p -8 p
Snacks:						
Water:						

Hits & Misses

What worked and what didn't? Why?

February

Sunday	Monday	Tuesday	Wednesday	Thursday	Friday	Saturday
	1	2	3	4	5	6
7	8	9	10	11	12	13
14	15	16	17	18	19	20
21	22	23	24	25	26	27
28						

WEEKLY GOALS!
1.
2.
3.
4.

WORKOUT SCHEDULE

	M	T	W	Th	F	S	S
Week 1	am pm	am pm	am pm	am pm	am pm	am pm	am pm
Week 2	am pm	am pm	am pm	am pm	am pm	am pm	am pm
Week 3	am pm	am pm	am pm	am pm	am pm	am pm	am pm
Week 4	am pm	am pm	am pm	am pm	am pm	am pm	am pm

Goal Tracker!

Weight	Non-scale Victories

Monthly Meal Planner

Grocery List

Meal Planning

Breakfast

1.
2.
3.
4.

Lunch

1.
2.
3.
4.

Dinner

1.
2.
3.
4.

Snacks

1.
2.
3.
4.

Meal Tracker

M	T	W	Th	F	S	S
6 a - 10 a	6 a - 10 a	6 a - 10 a	6 a - 10 a	6 a - 10 a	6 a - 10 a	6 a - 10 a
11 a - 2 p	11 a - 2 p	11 a - 2 p	11 a - 2 p	11 a - 2 p	11 a - 2 p	11 a - 2 p
3 p - 4 p	3 p - 4 p	3 p - 4 p	3 p - 4 p	3 p - 4 p	3 p - 4 p	3 p - 4 p
5 p -8 p	5 p -8 p	5 p -8 p	5 p -8 p	5 p -8 p	5 p -8 p	5 p -8 p
Snacks:						
Water:						

Hits & Misses

What worked and what didn't? Why?

March

Sunday	Monday	Tuesday	Wednesday	Thursday	Friday	Saturday
	1	2	3	4	5	6
7	8	9	10	11	12	13
14	15	16	17	18	19	20
21	22	23	24	25	26	27
28	29	30	31			

WEEKLY GOALS!
1.
2.
3.
4.

WORKOUT SCHEDULE

	M	T	W	Th	F	S	S
Week 1	am pm	am pm	am pm	am pm	am pm	am pm	am pm
Week 2	am pm	am pm	am pm	am pm	am pm	am pm	am pm
Week 3	am pm	am pm	am pm	am pm	am pm	am pm	am pm
Week 4	am pm	am pm	am pm	am pm	am pm	am pm	am pm

Goal Tracker!

Weight	Non-scale Victories

Monthly Meal Planner

Grocery List

Meal Planning

Breakfast

1.
2.
3.
4.

Lunch

1.
2.
3.
4.

Dinner

1.
2.
3.
4.

Snacks

1.
2.
3.
4.

Meal Tracker

M	T	W	Th	F	S	S
6 a - 10 a	6 a - 10 a	6 a - 10 a	6 a - 10 a	6 a - 10 a	6 a - 10 a	6 a - 10 a
11 a - 2 p	11 a - 2 p	11 a - 2 p	11 a - 2 p	11 a - 2 p	11 a - 2 p	11 a - 2 p
3 p - 4 p	3 p - 4 p	3 p - 4 p	3 p - 4 p	3 p - 4 p	3 p - 4 p	3 p - 4 p
5 p -8 p	5 p -8 p	5 p -8 p	5 p -8 p	5 p -8 p	5 p -8 p	5 p -8 p
Snacks:						
Water:						

Hits & Misses

What worked and what didn't? Why?

April

Sunday	Monday	Tuesday	Wednesday	Thursday	Friday	Saturday
				1	2	3
4	5	6	7	8	9	10
11	12	13	14	15	16	17
18	19	20	21	22	23	24
25	26	27	28	29	30	

WEEKLY GOALS!
1.
2.
3.
4.

WORKOUT SCHEDULE

	M	T	W	Th	F	S	S
Week 1	am pm	am pm	am pm	am pm	am pm	am pm	am pm
Week 2	am pm	am pm	am pm	am pm	am pm	am pm	am pm
Week 3	am pm	am pm	am pm	am pm	am pm	am pm	am pm
Week 4	am pm	am pm	am pm	am pm	am pm	am pm	am pm

Goal Tracker!

Weight	Non-scale Victories

Monthly Meal Planner

Grocery List

Meal Planning

Breakfast

1.
2.
3.
4.

Lunch

1.
2.
3.
4.

Dinner

1.
2.
3.
4.

Snacks

1.
2.
3.
4.

Meal Tracker

M	T	W	Th	F	S	S
6 a - 10 a	6 a - 10 a	6 a - 10 a	6 a - 10 a	6 a - 10 a	6 a - 10 a	6 a - 10 a
11 a - 2 p	11 a - 2 p	11 a - 2 p	11 a - 2 p	11 a - 2 p	11 a - 2 p	11 a - 2 p
3 p - 4 p	3 p - 4 p	3 p - 4 p	3 p - 4 p	3 p - 4 p	3 p - 4 p	3 p - 4 p
5 p -8 p	5 p -8 p	5 p -8 p	5 p -8 p	5 p -8 p	5 p -8 p	5 p -8 p
Snacks:						
Water:						

Hits & Misses

What worked and what didn't? Why?

May

Sunday	Monday	Tuesday	Wednesday	Thursday	Friday	Saturday
						1
2	3	4	5	6	7	8
9	10	11	12	13	14	15
16	17	18	19	20	21	22
23	24	25	26	27	28	29
30	31					

WEEKLY GOALS!
1.
2.
3.
4.

WORKOUT SCHEDULE

	M	T	W	Th	F	S	S
Week 1	am pm	am pm	am pm	am pm	am pm	am pm	am pm
Week 2	am pm	am pm	am pm	am pm	am pm	am pm	am pm
Week 3	am pm	am pm	am pm	am pm	am pm	am pm	am pm
Week 4	am pm	am pm	am pm	am pm	am pm	am pm	am pm

Goal Tracker!

Weight	Non-scale Victories

Monthly Meal Planner

Grocery List

Meal Planning

Breakfast

1.
2.
3.
4.

Lunch

1.
2.
3.
4.

Dinner

1.
2.
3.
4.

Snacks

1.
2.
3.
4.

Meal Tracker

M	T	W	Th	F	S	S
6 a - 10 a	6 a - 10 a	6 a - 10 a	6 a - 10 a	6 a - 10 a	6 a - 10 a	6 a - 10 a
11 a - 2 p	11 a - 2 p	11 a - 2 p	11 a - 2 p	11 a - 2 p	11 a - 2 p	11 a - 2 p
3 p - 4 p	3 p - 4 p	3 p - 4 p	3 p - 4 p	3 p - 4 p	3 p - 4 p	3 p - 4 p
5 p -8 p	5 p -8 p	5 p -8 p	5 p -8 p	5 p -8 p	5 p -8 p	5 p -8 p
Snacks:						
Water:						

Hits & Misses

What worked and what didn't? Why?

June

Sunday	Monday	Tuesday	Wednesday	Thursday	Friday	Saturday
		1	2	3	4	5
6	7	8	9	10	11	12
13	14	15	16	17	18	19
20	21	22	23	24	25	26
27	28	29	30			

WEEKLY GOALS!
1.
2.
3.
4.

WORKOUT SCHEDULE

	M	T	W	Th	F	S	S
Week 1	am pm	am pm	am pm	am pm	am pm	am pm	am pm
Week 2	am pm	am pm	am pm	am pm	am pm	am pm	am pm
Week 3	am pm	am pm	am pm	am pm	am pm	am pm	am pm
Week 4	am pm	am pm	am pm	am pm	am pm	am pm	am pm

Goal Tracker!

Weight	Non-scale Victories

Monthly Meal Planner

Grocery List

Meal Planning

Breakfast

1.
2.
3.
4.

Lunch

1.
2.
3.
4.

Dinner

1.
2.
3.
4.

Snacks

1.
2.
3.
4.

Meal Tracker

M	T	W	Th	F	S	S
6 a - 10 a	6 a - 10 a	6 a - 10 a	6 a - 10 a	6 a - 10 a	6 a - 10 a	6 a - 10 a
11 a - 2 p	11 a - 2 p	11 a - 2 p	11 a - 2 p	11 a - 2 p	11 a - 2 p	11 a - 2 p
3 p - 4 p	3 p - 4 p	3 p - 4 p	3 p - 4 p	3 p - 4 p	3 p - 4 p	3 p - 4 p
5 p -8 p	5 p -8 p	5 p -8 p	5 p -8 p	5 p -8 p	5 p -8 p	5 p -8 p
Snacks:						
Water:						

Hits & Misses

What worked and what didn't? Why?

July

Sunday	Monday	Tuesday	Wednesday	Thursday	Friday	Saturday
				1	2	3
4	5	6	7	8	9	10
11	12	13	14	15	16	17
18	19	20	21	22	23	24
25	26	27	28	29	30	31

WEEKLY GOALS!
1.
2.
3.
4.

WORKOUT SCHEDULE

	M	T	W	Th	F	S	S
Week 1	am pm	am pm	am pm	am pm	am pm	am pm	am pm
Week 2	am pm	am pm	am pm	am pm	am pm	am pm	am pm
Week 3	am pm	am pm	am pm	am pm	am pm	am pm	am pm
Week 4	am pm	am pm	am pm	am pm	am pm	am pm	am pm

Goal Tracker!

Weight	Non-scale Victories

Monthly Meal Planner

Grocery List

Meal Planning

Breakfast

1.
2.
3.
4.

Lunch

1.
2.
3.
4.

Dinner

1.
2.
3.
4.

Snacks

1.
2.
3.
4.

Meal Tracker

M	T	W	Th	F	S	S
6 a - 10 a	6 a - 10 a	6 a - 10 a	6 a - 10 a	6 a - 10 a	6 a - 10 a	6 a - 10 a
11 a - 2 p	11 a - 2 p	11 a - 2 p	11 a - 2 p	11 a - 2 p	11 a - 2 p	11 a - 2 p
3 p - 4 p	3 p - 4 p	3 p - 4 p	3 p - 4 p	3 p - 4 p	3 p - 4 p	3 p - 4 p
5 p -8 p	5 p -8 p	5 p -8 p	5 p -8 p	5 p -8 p	5 p -8 p	5 p -8 p
Snacks:						
Water:						

Hits & Misses

What worked and what didn't? Why?

August

Sunday	Monday	Tuesday	Wednesday	Thursday	Friday	Saturday
1	2	3	4	5	6	7
8	9	10	11	12	13	14
15	16	17	18	19	20	21
22	23	24	25	26	27	28
29	30	31				

WEEKLY GOALS!
1.
2.
3.
4.

WORKOUT SCHEDULE

	M	T	W	Th	F	S	S
Week 1	am pm	am pm	am pm	am pm	am pm	am pm	am pm
Week 2	am pm	am pm	am pm	am pm	am pm	am pm	am pm
Week 3	am pm	am pm	am pm	am pm	am pm	am pm	am pm
Week 4	am pm	am pm	am pm	am pm	am pm	am pm	am pm

Goal Tracker!

Weight	Non-scale Victories

Monthly Meal Planner

Grocery List

Meal Planning

Breakfast

1.
2.
3.
4.

Lunch

1.
2.
3.
4.

Dinner

1.
2.
3.
4.

Snacks

1.
2.
3.
4.

Meal Tracker

M	T	W	Th	F	S	S
6 a - 10 a	6 a - 10 a	6 a - 10 a	6 a - 10 a	6 a - 10 a	6 a - 10 a	6 a - 10 a
11 a - 2 p	11 a - 2 p	11 a - 2 p	11 a - 2 p	11 a - 2 p	11 a - 2 p	11 a - 2 p
3 p - 4 p	3 p - 4 p	3 p - 4 p	3 p - 4 p	3 p - 4 p	3 p - 4 p	3 p - 4 p
5 p -8 p	5 p -8 p	5 p -8 p	5 p -8 p	5 p -8 p	5 p -8 p	5 p -8 p
Snacks:						
Water:						

Hits & Misses

What worked and what didn't? Why?

September

Sunday	Monday	Tuesday	Wednesday	Thursday	Friday	Saturday
			1	2	3	4
5	6	7	8	9	10	11
12	13	14	15	16	17	18
19	20	21	22	23	24	25
26	27	28	29	30		

WEEKLY GOALS!
1.
2.
3.
4.

WORKOUT SCHEDULE

	M	T	W	Th	F	S	S
Week 1	am pm	am pm	am pm	am pm	am pm	am pm	am pm
Week 2	am pm	am pm	am pm	am pm	am pm	am pm	am pm
Week 3	am pm	am pm	am pm	am pm	am pm	am pm	am pm
Week 4	am pm	am pm	am pm	am pm	am pm	am pm	am pm

Goal Tracker!

Weight	Non-scale Victories

Monthly Meal Planner

Grocery List

Meal Planning

Breakfast

1.
2.
3.
4.

Lunch

1.
2.
3.
4.

Dinner

1.
2.
3.
4.

Snacks

1.
2.
3.
4.

Meal Tracker

M	T	W	Th	F	S	S
6 a - 10 a	6 a - 10 a	6 a - 10 a	6 a - 10 a	6 a - 10 a	6 a - 10 a	6 a - 10 a
11 a - 2 p	11 a - 2 p	11 a - 2 p	11 a - 2 p	11 a - 2 p	11 a - 2 p	11 a - 2 p
3 p - 4 p	3 p - 4 p	3 p - 4 p	3 p - 4 p	3 p - 4 p	3 p - 4 p	3 p - 4 p
5 p -8 p	5 p -8 p	5 p -8 p	5 p -8 p	5 p -8 p	5 p -8 p	5 p -8 p
Snacks:						
Water:						

Hits & Misses

What worked and what didn't? Why?

October

Sunday	Monday	Tuesday	Wednesday	Thursday	Friday	Saturday
					1	2
3	4	5	6	7	8	9
10	11	12	13	14	15	16
17	18	19	20	21	22	23
24	25	26	27	28	29	30
31						

WEEKLY GOALS!
1.
2.
3.
4.

WORKOUT SCHEDULE

	M	T	W	Th	F	S	S
Week 1	am pm	am pm	am pm	am pm	am pm	am pm	am pm
Week 2	am pm	am pm	am pm	am pm	am pm	am pm	am pm
Week 3	am pm	am pm	am pm	am pm	am pm	am pm	am pm
Week 4	am pm	am pm	am pm	am pm	am pm	am pm	am pm

Goal Tracker!

Weight	Non-scale Victories

Monthly Meal Planner

Grocery List

Meal Planning

Breakfast

1.
2.
3.
4.

Lunch

1.
2.
3.
4.

Dinner

1.
2.
3.
4.

Snacks

1.
2.
3.
4.

Meal Tracker

M	T	W	Th	F	S	S
6 a - 10 a	6 a - 10 a	6 a - 10 a	6 a - 10 a	6 a - 10 a	6 a - 10 a	6 a - 10 a
11 a - 2 p	11 a - 2 p	11 a - 2 p	11 a - 2 p	11 a - 2 p	11 a - 2 p	11 a - 2 p
3 p - 4 p	3 p - 4 p	3 p - 4 p	3 p - 4 p	3 p - 4 p	3 p - 4 p	3 p - 4 p
5 p -8 p	5 p -8 p	5 p -8 p	5 p -8 p	5 p -8 p	5 p -8 p	5 p -8 p
Snacks:						
Water:						

Hits & Misses

What worked and what didn't? Why?

November

Sunday	Monday	Tuesday	Wednesday	Thursday	Friday	Saturday
	1	2	3	4	5	6
7	8	9	10	11	12	13
14	15	16	17	18	19	20
21	22	23	24	25	26	27
28	29	30				

WEEKLY GOALS!
1.
2.
3.
4.

WORKOUT SCHEDULE

	M	T	W	Th	F	S	S
Week 1	am pm	am pm	am pm	am pm	am pm	am pm	am pm
Week 2	am pm	am pm	am pm	am pm	am pm	am pm	am pm
Week 3	am pm	am pm	am pm	am pm	am pm	am pm	am pm
Week 4	am pm	am pm	am pm	am pm	am pm	am pm	am pm

Goal Tracker!

Weight	Non-scale Victories

Monthly Meal Planner

Grocery List

Meal Planning

Breakfast

1.
2.
3.
4.

Lunch

1.
2.
3.
4.

Dinner

1.
2.
3.
4.

Snacks

1.
2.
3.
4.

Meal Tracker

M	T	W	Th	F	S	S
6 a - 10 a	6 a - 10 a	6 a - 10 a	6 a - 10 a	6 a - 10 a	6 a - 10 a	6 a - 10 a
11 a - 2 p	11 a - 2 p	11 a - 2 p	11 a - 2 p	11 a - 2 p	11 a - 2 p	11 a - 2 p
3 p - 4 p	3 p - 4 p	3 p - 4 p	3 p - 4 p	3 p - 4 p	3 p - 4 p	3 p - 4 p
5 p -8 p	5 p -8 p	5 p -8 p	5 p -8 p	5 p -8 p	5 p -8 p	5 p -8 p
Snacks:						
Water:						

Hits & Misses

What worked and what didn't? Why?

December

Sunday	Monday	Tuesday	Wednesday	Thursday	Friday	Saturday
			1	2	3	4
5	6	7	8	9	10	11
12	13	14	15	16	17	18
19	20	21	22	23	24	25
26	27	28	29	30	31	

WEEKLY GOALS!
1.
2.
3.
4.

WORKOUT SCHEDULE

	M	T	W	Th	F	S	S
Week 1	am pm	am pm	am pm	am pm	am pm	am pm	am pm
Week 2	am pm	am pm	am pm	am pm	am pm	am pm	am pm
Week 3	am pm	am pm	am pm	am pm	am pm	am pm	am pm
Week 4	am pm	am pm	am pm	am pm	am pm	am pm	am pm

Goal Tracker!

Weight	Non-scale Victories

Monthly Meal Planner

Grocery List

Meal Planning

Breakfast

1.
2.
3.
4.

Lunch

1.
2.
3.
4.

Dinner

1.
2.
3.
4.

Snacks

1.
2.
3.
4.

Meal Tracker

M	T	W	Th	F	S	S
6 a - 10 a	6 a - 10 a	6 a - 10 a	6 a - 10 a	6 a - 10 a	6 a - 10 a	6 a - 10 a
11 a - 2 p	11 a - 2 p	11 a - 2 p	11 a - 2 p	11 a - 2 p	11 a - 2 p	11 a - 2 p
3 p - 4 p	3 p - 4 p	3 p - 4 p	3 p - 4 p	3 p - 4 p	3 p - 4 p	3 p - 4 p
5 p -8 p	5 p -8 p	5 p -8 p	5 p -8 p	5 p -8 p	5 p -8 p	5 p -8 p
Snacks:						
Water:						

Hits & Misses

What worked and what didn't? Why?

Reference Guide

Here are some references for healthy recipes:

1. Pinterest
2. Kraftfoods.com
3. Goya.com
4. Allrecipes.com
5. Bettycrocker.com
6. Yummy.com
7. Delish.com
8. Foodnetwork.com
9. Epicurious.com
10. Myplate.gov

Serving Size Tips:

1. Protein: 1/2 C or Palm of hand, 2-3 servings per day
2. Fruit: 1/2 Cup = 1 serving, 2-4 servings per day
3. Vegetable: 1/2 Cup = 1 serving, 2-4 servings per day
4. Dairy: 1 Cup = 1 serving, 2-3 servings per day
5. Whole grains: 1/2 Cup = 1 serving, 6 servings per day

Don’t consume less than 1500 kcal per day.
3,500 kcal = 1lb

Made in United States
North Haven, CT
06 November 2026

21876161R10030